T0271771

"Losing a pregnancy or baby is often a shocking and de[vastating]
bereaved parents who are left not knowing how to grie[ve]
of the event. This journal provides a concrete way fo[r]
their feelings to words and make meaning of this traum[atic ...]
in twenty years of clinical practice, Rabinor's thoughtful prompts, practices,
and journal exercises invite these parents to reflect, process, and grieve their
loss(es), and begin to heal."

> —**Rayna D. Markin, PhD**, associate professor of counseling at
> Villanova University, in private practice at Attune Philadelphia
> Therapy Group, and author of *Psychotherapy for Pregnancy Loss*

"Rabinor has captured the essential elements to assist when grieving the
unspeakable loss of a baby in pregnancy or shortly after birth. As a therapist,
she uses the best techniques we know to guide the reader, utilizing the powerful
tool of journaling. Documenting the process and feelings, the reader feels truly
understood and supported with practices that validate this profound grief
experience. This journal is a must-have resource for clinicians and mourning
parents."

> —**Sharon N. Covington, LCSW-C**, Center for Reproductive Mental
> Health, editor of *Fertility Counseling*, and assistant clinical professor
> in the department of OB/GYN at Georgetown University School of
> Medicine

"Rabinor provides an excellent and comprehensive set of tools and exercises to
help process any type of reproductive loss in this book. It is well researched and
self-paced. I believe there is a richness in the loving-kindness used here which
could be used for many difficult life events."

> —**June Melin, MD, FACOG**, retired from thirty-three years of
> OB/GYN practice in San Diego, CA; physician and wellness
> committee member at Scripps Mercy Hospital in San Diego, CA;
> and medical board expert

"Rachel Rabinor has created an extremely useful work for anyone who has experienced a pregnancy loss. Readers are invited to use the journal in the fashion that suits them best. The strategies provide realistic and honest approaches to the process grieving individuals encounter, clearly recognizing there is no 'right' or 'wrong' way to experience grief or utilize the tools offered. Rabinor provides guidance to address aspects of healing, both internally and within the individual's social network."

—**William D. Petok, PhD**, clinical associate professor of obstetrics
and gynecology at Sidney Kimmel Medical College at Thomas
Jefferson University in Philadelphia, PA; and coeditor of *Psychological
and Medical Perspectives on Fertility Care and Sexual Health*

"This journal is an absolute must for anyone who has experienced pregnancy or baby loss. Rachel's warm and gentle language—combined with thoughtful journaling prompts, affirmations, and activities—provides a loving framework to honor reproductive loss and support healing. It beautifully articulates the multifaceted experiences many feel alone in, offering tangible strategies to guide the journaler. I will definitely be recommending this book to clients as a therapy companion."

—**Emily Remba, LCSW, PMH-C**, psychotherapist, and founder
and president of Reproductive Mental Health and Wellness

"This journal is a beautiful space to honor and grieve the loss of a child. Rabinor gives words to the complex emotions of losing a baby, while also offering a road map for grief and hope for healing. Rabinor's prompts, mantras, and exercises are comprehensive yet accessible for any stage of the grieving process. She offers compassion, wisdom, and a holding space, which is exactly what's needed during this overwhelming time."

—**Chelsea H. Sybrandt, LMFT**, maternal mental health therapist

"This is an invaluable resource for the unbearable grief and trauma of pregnancy and infant loss. In a society that is hardly built to support the 'normative' reproductive experiences, we are failing even more miserably to support those who endure loss and trauma. As a perinatal therapist specializing in loss, this journal includes much of what I do with patients in session—it serves as a trusted companion, guiding the individual through the multifaceted layers of grief and trauma; exploring, honoring, and nurturing one's expressions of grief; identifying boundary-setting with supports; and navigating how to move forward (not on)."

—**Tracy Gilmour-Nimoy, MS, LMFT, PMH-C**, psychotherapist, loss mom, and writer

The
Pregnancy &
Baby Loss
Guided Journal

Your Space to Process, Grieve & Heal
After Miscarriage, Stillbirth, or
Other Reproductive Loss

Rachel Rabinor, LCSW

New Harbinger Publications, Inc.

Publisher's Note

NEW HARBINGER PUBLICATIONS is a registered trademark of New Harbinger Publications, Inc.

New Harbinger Publications is an employee-owned company.

Copyright © 2024 by   Rachel Rabinor
New Harbinger Publications, Inc.
5720 Shattuck Avenue
Oakland, CA 94609
www.newharbinger.com

All Rights Reserved

The practice Butterfly Hug (pp. 10–11) was adapted from Jarero and Artigas 2023 ("The EMDR Therapy Butterfly Hug Method for Self-Administered Bilateral Stimulation." Research Gate. https://www.researchgate.net/publication/340280320), which is an EMDR method for self-administering bi-lateral stimulation.

Cover design by Amy Shoup

Interior design by Tom Comitta

Acquired by Ryan Buresh

Edited by Marisa Solis

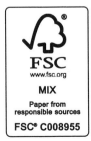

FSC
www.fsc.org
MIX
Paper from
responsible sources
FSC® C008955

Printed in the United States of America

26   25   24

10   9   8   7   6   5   4   3   2   1

First Printing

Contents

Foreword

"With the many unwelcome losses of life—of people, places, projects and possessions in seemingly endless succession, we are called on to reconstruct a world of meaning that has been challenged by loss, at every level from the simple habit structures of our daily lives, through our identities in a social world, to our personal and collective cosmologies, whether secular or spiritual." —Robert A. Neimeyer

Coping with grief and loss is part of the human condition. As painful as it is to lose a loved one, when it comes in the expected order—grandparents predeceasing parents, parents predeceasing children—we are able to grasp and ultimately accept it. But nothing prepares us for the loss of a pregnancy or baby. Expecting a life to begin, when suddenly faced with the unbelievable heartache of death, our dreams are shattered.

As a psychologist in the field of reproductive psychology, I have written extensively about the notion of the *reproductive story*, the sometimes conscious but largely unconscious narrative of what we expect life to be like as a parent. In this book, Rachel Rabinor has provided a tender and caring guide through the multitude of feelings people experience when their story has come to an unexpected, painful, and harshly abrupt ending.

The loss of a pregnancy or baby touches every aspect of life. Not only has your reproductive story gone awry, but you may also feel your body has betrayed you, you may blame yourself or your partner, you may feel enormous shame that everyone else can have a baby with ease, or you may feel alone and misunderstood. You may be feeling depressed, anxious, or angry with everyone and everything. Indeed, all that you thought you could count on may now be in question, from the most mundane to the spiritual. It's as if the rug has been pulled out from under you and everything in the room—from furniture to books to dishes—is precariously sailing through the air, and has yet to land. As agonizing as this is, these are normal reactions to the trauma of pregnancy or baby loss.

Sometimes people want and need to reach out to others as they process this loss, but sometimes people need time and space alone with their thoughts and feelings. This book can accompany you through dark and lonely moments. You can pick up this journal at any time, day or night, and find solace in its pages. Through exercises, affirmations, and prompts to help you reflect, this journal is designed to deepen your understanding of yourself.

In the midst of your reproductive trauma, it may feel as if all that stuff that is flying around in the air will never land again. This journal will not only assist you in putting the pieces of yourself and your world back together again, it will also help you write a new story for your future.

—Janet Jaffe, PhD

Introduction

Finding a way forward after a pregnancy or baby loss can feel impossible. You may feel stuck, out of control, or incredibly vulnerable. You may wonder how or why this happened to you. You might be suffering from an unidentified trauma and not realize it.

This journal is for anyone who carried their baby for any period of time and does not have them in their arms to hold. This journal is for you if you had a miscarriage. This journal is for you if you terminated a pregnancy for medical reasons. This journal is for you if you electively reduced a multiple pregnancy for maternal health conditions, psychological, or socioeconomic reasons. This journal is for you if your child was born still or sleeping. Regardless of the number of weeks or months you carried your baby, this journal is for you.

Pregnancy and baby loss are more common than we are led to believe. Miscarriage is estimated to impact 1 in 4 pregnancies; it is the most common complication of pregnancy. Stillbirth affects 1 in 160 pregnancies. For black women in the United States, these numbers are nearly double. Despite the frequency of pregnancy and baby loss, these devastating experiences are seldom talked about. Often, they result in feelings of unremitting sadness, depression, guilt, shame, and failure, which can lead to isolation and loneliness.

Why a Journal?

Navigating grief and the healing from loss can be a consuming process physically and emotionally. This journal offers a holding space. *Therapeutic journaling* is writing in response to feelings that may bubble up and may feel difficult to name. Research shows a consistent connection between therapeutic journaling and improved mental, emotional, and physical health. Putting your thoughts and feelings onto paper can offer you a new way to recognize complex feelings and process your grief.

This journal is designed to help you explore your feelings around this traumatic experience. You will process your emotions and develop strategies and insight for grieving, as you honor your story and gather strength to move on.

My Story

I, too, had the misfortune of navigating this path, sadly, more than once. I know the physical and emotional pain intimately. I am familiar with the accompanying despair, disappointment, and loneliness.

Twenty-two years ago I began graduate school at the Columbia University's School of Social Work in New York City. My first day of field training was September 11, 2001; needless to say, I was immersed in trauma, grief, and loss from day one.

Following graduation with a master's degree, I worked in pregnancy prevention for many years before making a 180° pivot to work with pregnant and parenting teens. Doing this work while experiencing my own transition to parenthood and reproductive traumas was a powerful influence on my career path. Postgraduate training in reproductive and perinatal mental health helped refine and further my expertise in the field.

In my private practice in San Diego, California, I specialize in supporting people who are striving to conceive, in mourning, or pregnant and parenting. I view my work through a trauma-informed lens and utilize evidence-based strategies to help clients alleviate suffering.

I wish I'd had this journal to guide me through my own grief process. Instead, I had pulled myself along through a cobbled-together network, largely derived from years of professional experience and extensive deep dives with everyone's best and worst friend—Google. Plus, a wonderful therapist. Now, it's an honor to bring my decades of experience to you here as you find your way forward.

Your reflections, along with the skills you learn and practice today, will serve you throughout your life. Please remember to be gentle and patient with yourself as you navigate your grief.

How to Use This Journal

This journal is broken into six parts covering the various ways in which pregnancy and baby loss impacts one's inner and outer worlds. Each part comprises four elements: prompts, practices, exercises, and affirmations. The structure is designed to help you reflect, process, and experiment with new strategies to grow through this challenging time. This journal will help you develop your innate resiliency as you heal from this heartbreaking loss.

That said, grief ebbs and flows. It doesn't follow a linear process; there is no specific place to begin or end. You may feel called to one part of the journal today and somewhere else tomorrow. You may need to take a break and come back a few days or weeks from now. There is no right way to grieve and no right way to heal or use this journal.

This journal is not a replacement for a therapist, medication, or medical treatment. It is a supportive guide to help you process a pregnancy or baby loss and a wide range of complicated feelings. However, if you are experiencing ongoing or debilitating feelings of depression or anxiety, I encourage you to consult a medical professional. Grief deserves your attention, and you may benefit from professional support in addition to the guidance of this journal.

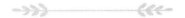

I am letting go of what I thought would happen
and learning to accept where I am.

Part I

Meet Yourself Where You Are

Experiencing a pregnancy or baby loss impacts one's mind, body, and spirit. You've been through a traumatic event and may still be reeling from the sudden news that's rocked your world, upending your hopes and dreams. It's not uncommon to feel shock and to struggle with accepting this new reality. Allowing yourself this space to reflect and process your loss is an important part of grieving.

While there is no universal timeline for grieving, making space to explore your thoughts, questions, fears, and emotions about your loss will help you develop compassion for yourself and where you are right now. Ultimately, journaling will help to move you forward, one day at a time.

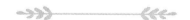

I am open to exploring this moment of suffering.

Recognizing Your Strength

Take a moment to acknowledge yourself for arriving here at this moment. You've bought and opened this book, a testament to your desire to heal. This takes courage. Feelings of sadness and helplessness may have led you to this journal, but it's also important to recognize the strength and dedication embedded in your actions.

What additional words of kindness can you offer yourself as you reflect on your decision to heal?

Your Connection to Your Baby

Attachment begins long before a confirmed pregnancy. Your hopes and dreams deepen as you envision yourself pregnant at an upcoming wedding, as you imagine your baby's first Halloween, or how you'll walk your child to the neighborhood school someday.

What were your earliest hopes when you learned of your pregnancy?

Remembering Your First Moments

What were the early days of your pregnancy like? Was your pregnancy planned or a surprise? Recall the exact moment you learned you were pregnant. Who was with you or who did you tell first? Reflect on your initial thoughts and feelings about this pregnancy.

_____

_____

_____

_____

_____

_____

_____

_____

_____

_____

_____

_____

_____

_____

_____

_____

_____

Your Reproductive Story

Long before conception, our reproductive dreams are born. Often this story begins in childhood, when visions of finding a partner and building a family become one with who we are and who we aspire to be—and ultimately shape our identity.

Dreaming about how many children you will have and what their sex and names will be are not uncommon. Imagining what sports they will play, or how they will excel in theater like you, or have your partner's green eyes, are all normal. Losing your sought-after baby was probably never part of your reproductive story.

Honoring and sharing your reproductive story can be a therapeutic part of the grieving process. Give yourself permission to write your story below. Share your earliest memories, hopes, and dreams of building your family. What kinds of plans did you have and how have these visions shifted over time?

Reflecting on Your Reproductive Story

What was it like to reflect on your reproductive story? Floating back in time and reconnecting with your younger self and your hopes and dreams can bring up a lot of emotions. Sometimes we recognize that our visions for the future were not just crafted from our own ideas but were influenced by our parents and grandparents, our friends, and the messages we've received from our larger spiritual communities as well as the media to which we've been exposed for decades.

What surprised you about your own reproductive story?

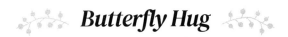

Butterfly Hug

Processing the trauma of a pregnancy or baby loss is exhausting physically and emotionally. The Butterfly Hug, which comes from eye movement desensitization and reprocessing (EMDR) therapy and is adapted here, can help you cope with symptoms of physical or emotional distress. What I like most about this practice is that you can do it anywhere, and you'll quickly notice the calming effects. Here's how to do it:

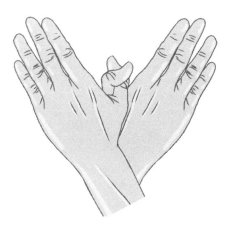

1. Make yourself comfortable: Stand, sit in a chair, or lie down, eyes open or closed.

2. Start by crossing your hands across your chest and hooking your thumbs to create the butterfly's body.

3. Allow your fingers (the butterfly wings) to rest just below your collarbone.

4. Locate the distress in your body and rate it from 0 (no distress) to 10 (the maximum distress you can feel).

5. Tap your left hand, then your right on your chest, alternating until you find a rhythm that feels good.

6. Breathe in and out through your nose and stop when you feel in your body that it has been enough.

7. Observe your body and notice any shifts in your distress.

If your distressing symptoms do not decrease, or they increase, consult an EMDR or other trauma therapist (see the Resources section at the end of this journal).

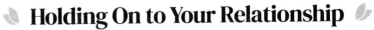 Holding On to Your Relationship

Even though your baby is gone, you don't have to let go of your relationship. This is part of your history. You may find comfort in celebrating your shared memories, however limited they may be. Had you selected a name for your baby? Perhaps you traveled somewhere special or you ate only ice cream and crackers while you carried your baby. Did you have a visit with friends that will forever remind you of this time? Which memories stand out for you? Honor these experiences and reminders.

Grieving takes time. I am patient with my healing process.

Identifying Symptoms of Grief

Take a moment to reflect on how you have been coping since your loss. Below are some common experiences for someone who's grieving. Circle any of the symptoms you've experienced since your loss.

Insomnia	Relationship challenges
Physical exhaustion	Clumsiness
Short attention span	Sleeping too much
Restlessness	Sleeping too little
Time loss	Nightmares
Confusion	Inability to cry
Hypersensitivity	Numbness
Phantom aches and pains	Anxiety
Sadness	Vivid or intense dreams
Anger	Loss of appetite

Eating too much

Loss of interest in activities

Feeling like you don't belong

Mood swings

Intense crying

Overwhelm or confusion with everyday tasks

Frustration

Feeling distanced from reality

Having a dark sense of humor

Crying silently

Screaming in the car

Feeling different from others

Outbursts that are tearful, angry, or the like

Loneliness

Memory loss

Physical pain

Tightness in throat or heaviness in chest

Reaching out to others

Withdrawing from others

Difficulty concentrating

Being short tempered

Reviewing the days and weeks leading up

Other _____

Other _____

🍃 Understanding Your Grief 🍃

You may have expected to cry and be sad. So maybe you've been caught off guard by some of the other emotions that pop up? All the reactions listed in the previous exercise are normal and often accompany a loss. Do any of them surprise you? Reflect on your grieving style thus far. What has startled or worried you?

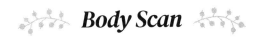

Body Scan

Grief is a full-body experience that impacts your thoughts, feelings, and physical sensations. Perhaps your body has been sending loud messages you can't possibly ignore. Or maybe you need to take a moment to listen carefully. This exercise is designed to help you listen to what your body's telling you. You may read the instructions all the way through first and then do the exercise; alternatively, you may access a free, guided audio recording at https://www.newharbinger.com/53868.

1. Find a comfortable position, seated or lying down.

2. Allow your eyes to close if it's comfortable to do so.

3. Take a few breaths. As you do, notice the weight of your body supported by the ground, the sofa, the chair, or wherever you are resting. Feel what it is like to rest your body as you breathe.

4. Bring your attention to the top of your head and scalp. Notice any throbbing, heat, tingling, or strong sensations, or nothing at all.

5. Lower your attention to your face... Scan your forehead, nose, jaw, and chin, and notice where tension may be stored. Allow the muscles to soften...

6. On the next out-breath, lower your focus to the neck. Letting the throat, back, and sides of the neck soften, notice any sensations on the surface of the skin or deeper within.

7. Continue in this slow, intentional way, scanning your body all the way down to your toes.

8. When you've finished, come back to this journal and reflect on your experience in the next prompt.

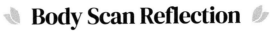 Body Scan Reflection

Reflect on your experience practicing the Body Scan exercise. What did you notice about your body? Was any area of your body calling for attention? How did those areas feel?

🍃 Living with Your Grief 🍃

Some people grieving a pregnancy or baby loss find comfort in doing—calling doctors, nurturing their body, or trying again. Others feel disconnected from their loss. And still others intentionally avoid all reference to the baby that once was, limiting exposure to pregnant people and any other reminders of their loss. What is it like to live with your grief?

It's okay to be angry at having to grieve.

Unanswered Questions About Your Loss

Losing a pregnancy or a baby can leave a lot of questions unanswered. Some may be tangible, others more existential. Like many, you may wonder why this happened or how you didn't know until it was too late. Maybe you're ruminating over what you could have done to stop it or how God or the higher powers that be could let something like this happen when you've been waiting for so long. You may be agonizing about the future.

Make a list below of any questions you still have about your loss or what that means for your future.

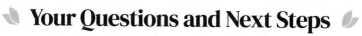# Your Questions and Next Steps

Review the list of questions that you wrote down in the previous exercise. Can they be answered by anyone in particular? If so, write their name or their profession (such as "MD" or "my rabbi") next to that question and make a plan to consult with these individuals. If the questions cannot be answered, reflect on what that feels like and what support you may need to move forward.

Self-Compassion Break

Self-compassion means treating yourself the way you'd treat a good friend. In the following practice, developed by psychologist Kristin Neff, you will engage in the three components of self-compassion: *mindfulness* (or the ability to nonjudgmentally notice what's happening for you now), *common humanity*, and *self-kindness*. You may read the instructions all the way through first and then do the exercise; alternatively, you may access a free, guided audio recording at https://www.newharbinger.com/53868.

1. Recall what you have gone through. Notice any stress or emotional discomfort in your body in this moment.

2. Now, say to yourself: **"This is a moment of suffering."** (That's practicing mindfulness.)

3. Acknowledge: **"Other people feel this pain too."** (That's acknowledging our common humanity.)

4. Now, put your hands over your heart and feel the warmth of your hands and the gentle touch of your hands on your chest.

5. Say to yourself: **"May I be kind to myself."** (That's engaging self-compassion.) Or ask yourself, "What do I need to hear right now to express kindness to myself?" Is there a phrase that speaks to you in your grief? Perhaps:

- *May I give myself the compassion that I need.*

- *May I forgive myself.*

- *May I be patient.*

This practice can be used any time of day or night and will help you remember to evoke the three aspects of self-compassion when you need them most.

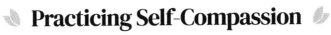 Practicing Self-Compassion

What does it feel like to comfort yourself in this way and realize that you can offer yourself kind words when you're struggling? Reflect on what it feels like when you put your hand on your heart, when you acknowledge your suffering and that of others, and when you offer yourself kind words.

Finding Meaning in Self-Compassion

Consider the three components of self-compassion—mindfulness, common humanity, and self-kindness. Which is most meaningful to you and important to acknowledge? Write about why this particular aspect is most powerful to you.

Part II

Leaning into Self-Love and Self-Care

Experiencing a pregnancy loss or losing your baby can cause you to feel powerless. It is often an all-consuming experience to process the physical loss while also navigating your internal emotional experience alongside the reactions of those around you. You may feel drained and unsure of the steps to move forward.

Self-love and self-care practices will help you begin to prioritize yourself and focus on offering yourself the best care possible as you heal from your loss. This part of the journal focuses on basic actions that are critical to reconnecting with and nourishing yourself as you move forward.

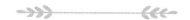

I'm doing the best I can right now and that is enough.

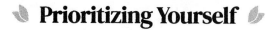 Prioritizing Yourself

When the world seems to be spinning out of control, prioritizing yourself is something tangible you can do while grieving. It may feel like you're wearing a weighted vest or slogging through a pool of molasses right now, but with small intentional acts you will begin to notice a shift.

What thoughts or words come up when you think about putting yourself first?

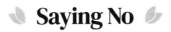 Saying No

While supportive relationships are valuable, setting boundaries after a loss can be an important step in prioritizing yourself. It can also help you feel in control when it seems as if so many things are out of your control. If you're someone who has struggled with setting boundaries in the past, it may feel difficult to set limits and say no.

Reflect on your experience setting boundaries prior to your pregnancy. In what areas have boundary setting been easy? Which have been more challenging? What thoughts and feelings come up when you think of setting boundaries now?

Understanding Boundaries

Some people hesitate to set boundaries for fear of rejection or of being unloved. They assume boundaries will threaten closeness and connection. This is paradoxical thinking, however. Dr. Brené Brown, a social work researcher, teaches that compromising your true self in an effort to find belonging and connection will leave you feeling lonelier with people than you would have been if you'd remained true to yourself.

If you have a habit of saying yes when you really want to say no, think about a looming commitment you've made to someone that you'd like to skip. Dig into what your true needs are.

1. If you say or have said yes, is it because of something you want from the person, such as approval or to fit in? Or are you doing it to please them?

   _____

   _____

   _____

2. Do you struggle to feel deserving of getting your needs met or of feeling worthy?

   _____

   _____

   _____

3. Ask yourself how you want to feel and what emotions you most want to have. Ask yourself how accepting this invitation or saying yes is going to make you feel.

_____

_____

_____

4. Now, ask yourself how turning down the invitation or saying no is going to make you feel.

_____

_____

_____

Setting New Boundaries

Make a commitment to limit your exposure to people or places that may be triggering. Unfollow friends or influencers related to pregnancy on social media. Practice saying no. No, you don't need to go to a baby shower. No, you don't need to go to dinner with friends when someone is pregnant or you just don't feel like talking about your loss.

What boundaries can you give yourself permission to set?

Identifying Your Core Values

If setting boundaries continues to feel difficult, reflect on your *core values*. Values are your deepest desires for how you want to live and behave as a human being.

This exercise is modified from acceptance and commitment therapy. Using the list below, circle your top ten values. Next, rate them from 1 to 10, with 1 representing the value that is most important to you in your life right now. From there, you will see your top three values naturally emerge. Put a star next to them.

Accepting	Courageous
Adventurous	Creative
Assertive	Curious
Authentic	Efficient
Caring	Empathic
Committed	Engaged
Compassionate	Fair
Cooperative	Friendly

Forgiving	Respectful
Fun-loving/humorous	Responsible
Generous	Self-caring
Genuine	Sincere
Grateful	Supportive
Helpful	Trusting
Honest	Trustworthy
Kind	Other _____
Loving	Other _____
Mindful	Other _____
Open	Other _____
Playful	
Reliable	

Living in Alignment with Your Values

Setting boundaries and developing self-care practices will help you live a more meaningful life—and one that's more aligned with your values and supportive of your healing.

Reflecting on the values you've identified, what is one thing you can do to live in greater alignment with those values? How will you incorporate that thing in your life?

I am discovering new strengths within myself.

🌿 Pain vs. Suffering 🌿

Pain tells us that something is wrong. It's a normal, healthy response when we lose a baby; it's something we can't avoid or control. *Suffering*, on the other hand is the story we tell ourselves about the pain. It's the thoughts, judgments, and beliefs about our pain that make it feel worse.

What are some of the behaviors, thoughts, or stories linked to your suffering? Examples might include not getting enough food; surrounding yourself with unhelpful, dismissive, or exhausting people; self-blame; suppressing your feelings; or intrusive thoughts about loss and grief that keep cycling through your mind. Think about anything that depletes, exhausts, or aggravates you beyond the pain of your loss.

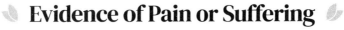 Evidence of Pain or Suffering

To reduce suffering, we need to recognize what it looks like to suffer and also what it looks like to do well. *Share some of the signs you've noticed that indicate you are doing well or suffering.* An example of doing well might be sleeping through the night, whereas insomnia may be a sign of suffering.

Doing Well	Suffering

What Activities Help Reduce Suffering?

Let's look a bit deeper. What are some of the things that contribute to you doing well? If your loss was recent, you may find this difficult. Try thinking about moments when your grief lessened. Did your friend bring over your favorite meal? Maybe you took a walk in the park? Did a friend or relative share a personal loss or moment of grief with you?

Think back over the past few days or weeks and try to identify five or more moments when you felt a break from or a lessening of the pain.

1.

2.

3.

4.

5.

Visualization

Visualization helps you prepare for and practice responding to a situation before it happens. This can lead to a decrease in overall stress. It also helps you achieve your goals as you allow your brain to see, hear, and feel the success in your mind. You may read the instructions all the way through first and then do the exercise; alternatively, you may access a free, guided audio recording at https://www.newharbinger.com/53868.

Take a moment to close your eyes. Visualize yourself doing or asking for one of the five activities you identified in the previous prompt. Imagine tomorrow that you're able to re-create one of those experiences. Notice what you see in front of you, behind you, above you, and beneath your feet. Notice the sounds, the smells. What does it feel like to be in that moment, having a break from the pain? Notice what that feels like in your body. Allow all those good feelings to spread throughout your body. Sit with those sensations as you breathe and just notice how it feels to have a moment when things feel okay.

🍃 Committing to Self-Care 🍃

Think about your healing and the goals you have for your future self. List thirty things you can do that prioritize your self-care and show self-love. Petting your dog or cat, eating a bowl of ice cream, taking a walk, declining an invitation, asking for help, taking time off work, taking a break from social media, and reaching out to a therapist are a few ideas.

Commit to doing one thing from your list each day for the next month. You may even benefit from repeating the same five to ten things. Do what works for you. And if you miss a day or two or three, use that as an opportunity to practice self-compassion.

1. _____

2. _____

3. _____

4. _____

5. _____

6. _____

7. _____

8. _____

9. _____

10. _____

11. _____

12.

13.

14.

15.

16.

17.

18.

19.

20.

21.

22.

23.

24.

25.

26.

27.

28.

29.

30.

How Self-Compassionate Am I?

Self-compassion can help to increase happiness, self-confidence, physical health, and life satisfaction. It can also decrease feelings of depression, anxiety, stress, and shame. Let's test your self-compassion using a modified version of Kristin Neff's Self-Compassion Scale.

Read each statement carefully and then write down the number, using the scale from 1 to 5, that best describes how often the behavior is true for you.

Almost Never			Almost Always	
1	2	3	4	5

1. I try to be understanding and patient toward those aspects of my personality I don't like.

2. When something painful happens, I try to take a balanced view of the situation.

3. I try to see my failings as part of the human condition.

4. When I'm going through a very hard time, I give myself the caring and tenderness I need.

5. When something upsets me, I try to keep my emotions in balance.

6. When I feel inadequate in some way, I try to remind myself that feelings of inadequacy are shared by most people.

7. When I fail at something important to me, I become consumed by feelings of inadequacy.

8. When I'm feeling down, I tend to feel like most other people are probably happier than I am.

9. When I fail at something that's important to me, I tend to feel alone in my failure.

10. When I'm feeling down, I tend to obsess and fixate on everything that's wrong.

11. I'm disapproving and judgmental about my own flaws and inadequacies.

12. I'm intolerant and impatient toward those aspects of my personality I don't like.

What your score may mean:

Total (sum of all 12 items) = _____

Mean score (total divided by 12) = _____

What your score may mean:

1 to 2.5 indicates that you are low in self-compassion

2.5 to 3.5 indicates you are moderate in self-compassion

3.5 to 5.0 indicates you are high in self-compassion

Responding with Self-Compassion

Don't worry if you scored lower in self-compassion than you would like. This quiz isn't another excuse to beat yourself up. Instead, use it as a gentle way to increase your awareness of the aspects of self-compassion that are difficult for you. Fortunately, self-compassion is a skill that can be learned. What are some words of compassion you can offer yourself to honor where you are right now?

With or without a baby, I am worthy.

Becoming Self-Compassionate Through Mindfulness

Developing compassion for yourself starts with mindfulness. Tuning in to where you are right now and noticing your suffering is a necessary step before you can learn to respond with kindness. Acknowledging your pain, your thoughts, and physical sensations without judgment is a practice.

The goal of mindfulness is not to have no thoughts or distractions. Rather, it is to notice these normal events and practice responding to them— and yourself—compassionately. Here are steps for a simple mindfulness practice:

1. Commit to do this practice for three minutes. Note your start time on a clock but do not set an alarm.

2. Take a few breaths as you settle in.

3. Allow your eyes to close or gaze softly at the ground.

4. Notice your breath as you breathe in and out.

5. If you notice your mind has started wandering, guide it back to your breath. If you notice a critical or judgmental voice chastising you for losing focus, just notice it and bring your mind back to your breath.

6. If you stop before the three minutes, just close your eyes again, remember to be compassionate with yourself, and continue until the three minutes is over. When you've finished, come back to this journal and reflect on your experience in the next prompt.

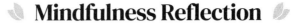 Mindfulness Reflection

A mindfulness practice is designed to give you the mental space to pause, so you're able to choose how you'd like to respond. In that pause, you can ask yourself what you need, and in response you can give yourself the comfort and support you desire.

Write about your experience with the three-minute mindfulness exercise on the previous page. What thoughts came up? How did you respond? How did it feel?

⁓ *I'm Proud Of...* ⁓

Losing a baby can cause feelings of insecurity and self-doubt. As an antidote, we may need to cultivate greater self-love. This happens by recognizing our strengths and positive qualities, and tapping into the essence of what makes you unique and proud to be you.

List five positive qualities that describe you. For each one, give evidence. For example, if "being loving toward others" is one of your qualities, you might write, "I make it a priority to show my partner love each day. For example, yesterday I made their favorite dinner."

1. _____

_____

2. _____

_____

3. _____

_____

4. _____

_____

5. _____

_____

Constructive Rest

The psoas, the muscle group that connects our spine and legs, is one of the most important muscles connected to our emotions. Emotional trauma or an ongoing lack of emotional support can lead to a chronically contracted psoas. This pose is a passive way to release tension in the psoas.

Plan to hold this position for ten to twenty minutes. You may want to listen to soothing music or nature sounds to help you relax.

1. Resting on your back, bend your knees and place feet on the floor parallel to each other, hip-width apart.

2. Place your heels twelve to sixteen inches from your buttocks.

3. Place a folded towel or a book under your head.

4. Keep your arms below shoulder height, letting them rest over the ribcage, to the sides of your body, or on your belly.

5. There is nothing to do; just be. The psoas is released by the movement of your breath and by gravity.

6. When you've finished, come back to this journal and reflect on your experience in the next prompt.

If your legs are uncomfortable or you can't fully relax, try repositioning your legs so that your calves are resting on the seat of a chair or couch.

Reflecting on Constructive Rest

Taking care of your mind and body can sometimes feel like just another thing to do. The beauty of the Constructive Rest pose is that it's just the opposite.

What was it like to just be and know that you're nourishing both your emotional and physical health? What thoughts or feelings come up when you think about letting yourself rest? How likely are you to try this again?

Part III

Make Space for Your Emotions

Your grief may feel inescapable. The basic acts of finding focus and making decisions may be chores now, never mind working or caring for other children. The complexity of your emotions may make it feel easier to disconnect and isolate yourself.

However, making time and space for your shifting emotions takes courage and is an important step in healing. Your emotional health deserves your attention, especially during this heart-wrenching time. Regardless of other losses you've faced, this is a new and unique grief you are suffering. Your story matters. Your loss matters. You matter.

This part of this journal will explore your emotional experience and provide strategies and tools for coping.

→》》——————《《←

I give myself time and space to feel all my feelings.

Early Emotional Experiences

Many of us have learned that being emotional is a weakness, and in turn we learned to ignore or avoid our feelings. Yet, feelings are signals from our body that can help us understand ourselves and make good decisions. For example, feeling fear when crossing a busy street in traffic helps us stay safe.

Reflect on your comfort identifying and communicating your emotions. What messages did you receive from your caregivers growing up about emotions or being emotional? How has this impacted you today?

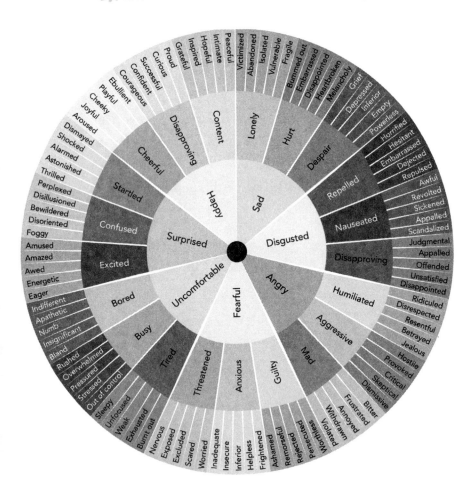

Most adults can name only three emotions: happiness, sadness, and anger. But according to a UCLA study, increasing your vocabulary around emotions allows you to better recognize and manage emotional experiences. It also means you can better communicate your needs and get support from others. When you name your emotions or thoughts, you can tame your physical response too, according to Dr. Dan Siegel.

Using the wheel of emotions, name the emotions you are feeling right now. Do they cluster around one core emotion, or are they evenly dispersed? Make an expansive list of emotions you've experienced since your loss.

Feeling Your Emotions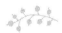

Note one of the more challenging emotions from the Name It to Tame It exercise that you've been struggling with. See if you can observe where you experience this emotion in your body. You may have an urge to avoid this feeling; instead, see if you can push yourself to experience it. How long can you sit with discomfort? Be gentle; it may take time to practice sensing your emotions.

After your first practice, write about your experience.

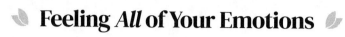 Feeling *All* of Your Emotions

It may feel complicated to focus on feelings other than sorrow or anger right now. From the emotions you identified in the Name It to Tame It exercise, choose one that is close to happy. Think about your most recent experience feeling joyful. Where do you experience this feeling in your body? Do you welcome the sensation or try to suppress it? Give yourself a moment to linger with feeling joy and write about the experience.

Expressive Journaling

Pregnancy and baby loss bring up a host of complicated feelings. It can be hard to hold two or more seemingly opposing emotions, like relief and sadness or guilt and anger, at the same time. Yet, routinely writing down your thoughts and feelings—which you have been doing in this journal—can help you recognize complex feelings and process your grief. If you'd like to try an experiment with expressive writing, based on research by James Pennebaker, the following steps can guide you:

1. **Carve out time.** Aim for fifteen minutes four days in a row.

2. **Experiment with your method.** Handwrite, use a phone or computer, or record yourself speaking.

3. **Find the right place.** Where you write can affect your feelings. Should it be quiet? With music? Inside? Outside? You might have to experiment to find the right place for you.

4. **Don't edit yourself.** Access your feelings and allow yourself to flow. Leave out the punctuation; make mistakes! The goal is self-expression, not perfection!

5. **Reread.** Your writing is a record of your life. Go back and see what you've written. You may want to rewrite it or you may want to rip it up. Your choice!

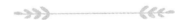

I may feel as if I will fall apart if I allow all my emotions to come out, and that's okay.

I'm Feeling…

Identifying our emotions allows us to become curious about what we need in a given moment. And practicing mindful awareness and learning to recognize our thoughts and feelings, no matter how difficult or uncomfortable they may be, builds confidence that we can handle painful experiences.

Notice what happens as you focus on how you're feeling in this moment. If you hear yourself say, "I think…," pause and go deeper to identify your emotion, asking what it is you're *feeling*. Throughout the next few days, practice noticing your feelings. Come back to this journal and share any observations about noticing the feelings beneath your thoughts.

I'm feeling

I'm feeling

I'm feeling

I'm feeling

I'm feeling

❧ Understanding Your Worries ❧

Worry is a natural feeling after losing a baby. You may be worried that something you did or didn't do contributed to your loss. You might be worrying about what the future holds: *Will I get pregnant again? Will I experience another loss? How will I survive another loss?*

Share your worries. After you're finished writing, note whether the worries are in the past (label with a P) or in the future (label with a F).

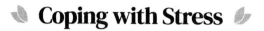 Coping with Stress

When we experience an unexpected stressor or trauma such as a pregnancy or baby loss, the brain's limbic system is fired up and releases adrenaline and cortisol. The flood of these hormones may cause you to freeze up, act out, or shut down—activating your body's fight, flight, or freeze response.

Reflect on how you've responded to your loss. Are you feeling stuck in your body—cold, numb, stiff—with restricted breathing? Do you have a sense of impending dread (freeze)? Have you noticed tightness in your jaw or fists and a desire to physically kick or punch, with feelings of anger or rage (fight)? Or are you finding it hard to focus or feeling anxious, trapped, tense, or restless (flight)? How has your reaction to your loss shifted in the days, weeks, or months since it first happened?

4:8 Breathing Practice

It's anxiety-producing to think and rethink the details of your traumatic loss. Anticipating what will happen next can be equally distressing. Spending excessive time worrying about past or future situations is exhausting and rarely brings relief.

Instead, try staying in the present moment. This breathing technique stimulates the *vagus nerve*, which regulates your heart, digestive system, and breathing rate. When the vagus nerve is activated, it will temper your physiological stress response, resulting in a feeling of calm, which will help you stay in the moment.

1. To begin, sit still and tall somewhere comfortable. Close your eyes and begin breathing through your nose.

2. Inhale for a count of 4.

3. Exhale for a count of 8.

4. Keep your breathing even and smooth. If the 4:8 count feels too long, try decreasing the exhale to a count of 7, or 6 if needed. The most important thing is that the exhale is longer than the inhale.

5. Continue for at least three minutes. Notice how you feel physically and mentally.

Understanding Guilt and Self-Blame

It's not uncommon to feel guilty or responsible for your loss. Questions like *Was it what I ate? What I didn't eat? Was it the exercise or the drink I had?* can percolate. In reality, there may not be answers as to why this happened, and such thoughts unnecessarily induce self-blame.

Recognizing the self-defeating power of these thoughts can help you let go of them. Write about how you've experienced guilt or self-blame since your loss, including whether you've felt guilty for experiencing emotions of joy or pleasure. If you were able to let those thoughts go, how did you do it, and how did it impact your feelings?

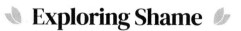 Exploring Shame

Shame and guilt are often confused, both of which can delay your healing. According to Brené Brown, a specialist in shame research, *guilt* is the feeling "I did something bad" while *shame*, bound by stigma and silence, is the feeling that "I am bad."

The cultural silence around baby loss can send messages that one has failed in their duty to keep their baby safe, or they are selfish or a bad person for terminating for medical reasons. After all, if people aren't talking about it, it must be something to be ashamed of and therefore hidden from others. Processing beliefs of shame and feelings of guilt can reduce the heavy weight many continue to carry despite weeks and months of mourning. How has shame impacted your healing?

Acknowledging Your Anger

Anger is an understandable reaction to losing your baby. You may feel angry at medical providers, at friends and family for how they did or didn't respond, or simply at those who have been fortunate to easily conceive and carry a healthy baby to term.

Recognizing thoughts that provoke anger and finding ways to challenge them will bring positive change. Can you recognize any recent triggering thoughts and ways you have successfully coped with anger?

Normalizing Feelings of Failure, Jealousy, and Loneliness

It may feel uncomfortable to feel envy or jealousy toward friends or strangers for their pregnancies. You might question your worth, deeming your loss a personal failure and believing that you are responsible. Unshared, these common feelings can cause loneliness, isolation, and potentially depression.

How does it feel to know that these are common reactions to losing a baby? And how does it feel to think about sharing them?

My heart is big enough to hold everything I feel.

Letter to a Friend or Loved One

Some people struggle with offering themselves tender care and compassion. If that sounds like you, try to put that part of yourself aside while you participate in this exercise. Imagine your cousin, sibling, or best friend is grieving a similar loss. What would you tell them? How would you respond to them when they tell you they feel guilty or to blame? Write a letter to your loved one offering the support you think they deserve.

❧ Reflecting on Your Letter ❧

Developing self-compassion is a crucial practice to support your healing. It doesn't happen overnight and requires regular effort. With that in mind, reflect on your letter to a friend or loved one from the previous exercise and what you have learned about the way you talk to *yourself* compared with how you would talk to *someone you care for*. Then, try to write a similar compassionate letter to yourself.

Waves of Emotion

Our thoughts, like the ocean, are always moving, rising and falling. Mindfulness teaches us to notice our thoughts, feelings, and emotions; acknowledge them; and let them go as we return to the present moment without judging or clinging to them. Practicing mindfulness regularly teaches that emotions come and go, like waves in the sea. Occasionally a big wave in the form of an intense thought or feeling can hook our minds and take us on a ride.

Over time, with practice, you can notice these thoughts as well and watch them come and go. Follow these steps for a basic mindfulness practice, refer to the mindfulness meditation recommendations in the Resources at the end of this journal, or access a free, guided audio recording at https://www.newharbinger.com/53868.

1. Sit in a comfortable but upright position.

2. Begin to tune in to your breath, noticing the cool air as you breathe in and the warm air as you breathe out.

3. Throughout the meditation, notice any thoughts that come up, noting them as "thinking" or "a thought." Then, bring your attention back to the breath.

4. Come back to your breath whenever you realize your mind has drifted away. This might happen dozens of times, and that's okay!

Emotions Come and Go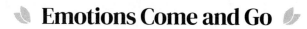

There is nothing easy about navigating the roller coaster of emotions that comes after a traumatic loss. The grief you feel may lessen, but it will likely never go away completely. There will be reminders and anniversaries that stir up emotions. Some days will be harder. Others won't feel quite so raw.

Reflect on the emotional waves of your experience. How have you experienced the ebb and flow of your feelings? Does the Waves of Emotion practice on the previous page help to normalize your experience?

Part IV

Reconnect with Your Body

The shock and devastation of losing a pregnancy or a baby can be traumatic, affecting both the physical and emotional self. Trauma is stored in the body, often presenting as physical pain or discomfort. Emotionally, you may have complicated feelings about your body right now.

As you move through this part of the journal, you may find emotional pain surface, whether from this recent traumatic loss or a history of trauma. Please consider additional support from a licensed therapist trained in reproductive mental health and trauma. Resources are available at the end of this journal. Treating your body with kindness and compassion is essential as you rebuild the relationship between your emotional and physical self.

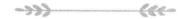

I love and accept myself the way I am.

✿ Are You in Your Body? ✿

Your body may be a continual reminder of your loss. You may respond by distancing yourself from your body in order to avoid feeling and to suppress the trauma memory. *Post-traumatic stress responses* may include shallow breathing, racing heart, pain, fatigue, and headaches, among many others. These physical reactions can interfere with healing after trauma.

Using a deep-breathing exercise can help you reconnect to your body. How have you distanced yourself from your body? What comes up for you as you think about reconnecting or strengthening the connection with your body?

Befriending Your Body Again

Your body has been through a physical trauma and now it's returning or has returned to its pre-pregnancy shape. Taking care of your body means tuning in to your body's sensations, which may provide new information.

It may be confusing to know if what's happening to your body after a pregnancy loss or stillbirth is normal, or if you should seek medical attention. Here, for reference, are some of the typical symptoms following a pregnancy loss:

- Mild cramping (for a few days)

- Nausea

- Diarrhea

- Light bleeding or spotting for up to six weeks

- Breast discomfort or engorgement, or leaking milk

Here are some other potential experiences in pregnancy loss to be aware of:

- Vaginal bleeding, similar to a menstrual period, should stop after one week.

- Depending on your menstrual cycle, normal periods should resume in three to six weeks after breast milk production has stopped.

- Lower abdominal pain, similar to menstrual cramps, should cease after a few days.

- Some pregnancy hormones can remain in the blood for up to two months after a loss.

Again, if you have any concerns about whether what you're experiencing is normal, don't be afraid to seek medical attention.

Felt Sense

The *felt sense* is a term coined by philosopher Eugene Gendlin of the International Focusing Institute. It's a combination of emotion, awareness, intuitiveness, and embodiment. This exercise offers an opportunity to gain greater awareness of the felt sense. You will need colored pencils, pens, crayons, or markers.

Using the body map, color the areas of the body where you presently sense discomfort, pain, tightness, or tension. Select colors that represent the type of sensation you are feeling in a particular part of the body. Think about the type of pressure and the strokes you use to best reflect the sensations in those parts of the body. After completing the body map, label the colored areas with emotions. Then write any observations you have about your body map and this process.

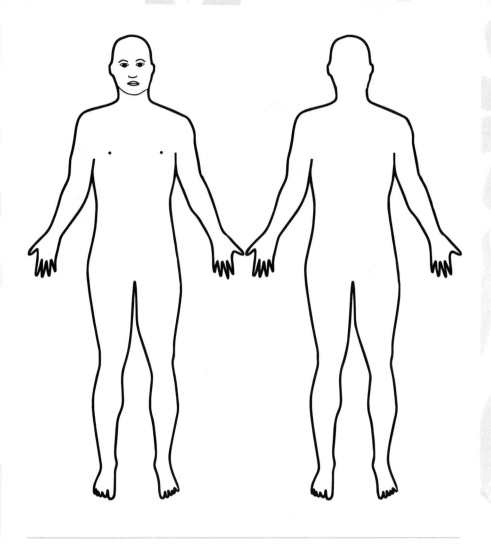

❧ Your Changing Body ☙

You may have struggled to accept the changes that initially came with pregnancy, and now you may be challenged to accept the changes that you must adjust to after your loss. Perhaps you started to gain weight and began wearing maternity clothes that you will hold onto, even though you're no longer pregnant. Or maybe you lost weight due to morning sickness.

What thoughts and feelings about your body has your loss triggered or unearthed? Remember, naming our feelings helps us accept them and offers ourselves compassion during this heartbreaking time.

Your Relationship with Your Body

You may feel as if your body has failed you. You may have felt a deep connection to your body during pregnancy and were motivated to care for it in new ways in support of your baby—nourishing yourself with sleep, exercise, and healthy food. When you've developed feelings of pride at your ability to become pregnant and carry your baby, a pregnancy loss can feel like a betrayal.

How has your pregnancy and loss affected your connection to your body?

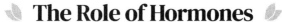 The Role of Hormones

Estrogen and progesterone rise during pregnancy and then decline after a pregnancy or baby is lost. This shift can affect your mental and emotional state, triggering feelings of sadness and hopelessness, as well as fatigue, changes in mood, and sluggishness. The risk of depression increases during major life events or transitions like this. Hormones may intensify the feelings you already experience due to the grief of your loss. Understanding the connection between hormones and your moods may help you be more self-accepting.

How have you navigated the shift of hormones since your loss?

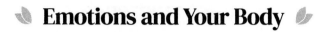 Emotions and Your Body

Emotions are often connected with certain body areas. A lump in your throat or a pit in your stomach may signal fear. An expansion in your chest may signal pride. Suppressing your emotions can lead to physical stress on your body, high blood pressure, memory challenges, decreased self-esteem, aggression, anxiety, and depression. Long-term physical impacts of suppressed emotions may include diabetes and heart disease. Understanding the mind-body connection is an important part of caring for your body.

As you scan your body now, do you have a sense that certain emotions are causing physical symptoms? If your body could talk, what would it say?

I am inherently worthy as a person.

Your Experience

Depending how far along you were in your pregnancy, you may have been offered one or more of these treatment options: medication management such as misoprostol; dilation and curettage (D&C); expectant management whereby you waited for the body to naturally expel the tissue; dilation and evacuation (D&E); or an induction followed by vaginal delivery.

Or perhaps your loss was a complete surprise, and you unexpectedly miscarried or delivered a baby that was born still. The intense grief and overwhelm of making decisions, or of having no decisions to make, may have left you in a state of shock.

Take your time to process the physical and emotional experience you endured. Feel free to come back to this tomorrow, next week, or next month—whenever you feel ready to share.

RAIN

RAIN is a four-step structured mindfulness and self-compassion practice. Originally developed by Michele McDonald, this version, modified by Dr. Tara Brach, is effective for working with intense or difficult emotions. However, instead of focusing on the thoughts in your mind, allow your body to do the work. As you work through the four steps, ask yourself, *What does it really feel like in my body to feel the way I feel? What if I allowed this feeling to unfold, without judging or censoring?* I recommend using the free, guided audio recording provided at https://www.newharbinger. com/53868, or refer to the Resources for other suggestions.

RAIN is an acronym for the four steps of the process. Go through these steps when you are feeling intense or difficult emotions rise:

> Recognize what is happening. What's going on inside of you? What are your physical sensations, emotions, thoughts, feelings? Identify what is happening in the present moment, such as, "I'm feeling overwhelmed; I don't know what our next step is and everyone keeps asking how they can help."

> Allow things to be just as they are. Allowing the thoughts, emotions, feelings, or sensations recognized to just be there doesn't mean you have to like the situation.

> Investigate the emotions you've recognized. Become curious about them and how they feel in your body. Notice how the feelings are affecting you.

Nurture yourself. Pinpoint what you need in this moment. Perhaps it is gentle words of comfort that you can offer yourself. Or healthy meals you ask a friend to deliver to your front door. Who can fulfill your needs?

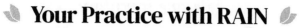 Your Practice with RAIN

After practicing RAIN, what do you notice? Did you experience any shifts within? Do you feel lighter, calmer, or more relaxed in your body?

Lifestyle Inventory

Caring for yourself may be difficult to prioritize while grieving. Challenges falling or staying asleep, changes in appetite, and fluctuations of mood can impact your overall wellness. Take an inventory of where you are regarding the following areas of health. Write about their quality, quantity, and anything else that comes to mind.

Exercise

_____

_____

Sleep

_____

_____

Diet

_____

_____

Relaxation

_____

_____

Spirituality

_____

_____

Smoking

_____

_____

Alcohol

_____

_____

Tobacco

_____

_____

Caffeine

_____

_____

Vitamins or supplement

_____

_____

Water

_____

_____

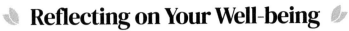

Reflecting on Your Well-being

What did you learn about yourself after completing the lifestyle inventory? Which areas of your health could benefit from change? Choose three areas from the inventory; for each, name one small adjustment you could make to improve your physical health. Consider how you would feel if you were to make those slight changes for a week, then a month.

I take care of myself as I heal.

Assessing Your Eating Habits

Recall how you have been eating the last few days. Are there times when you rushed a meal? Ate a relaxed meal? Forgotten to eat? What do you notice about your eating patterns related to your overall mood and physical energy?

_____

_____

_____

_____

_____

_____

_____

_____

_____

_____

_____

Sleep Hygiene

Sleep hygiene is a fancy way of saying "sleep health." Getting ample sleep is key to a full recovery. Think about your sleep habits historically. Are you a person who requires nine hours a night to function, or is five sufficient? What is your before-bed routine like? Do you do the same things to help you return to sleep when you wake up in the middle of the night? How have your sleep habits changed through your pregnancy and loss?

Visualizing Wellness

A healthy diet and ample sleep are critical for recovery from a traumatic experience. Trauma responses often lead to either a decrease in appetite or increase in cravings for comfort food—sugary, salty, fatty foods. The short-term benefit is that these foods increase certain neurotransmitters that release hormones and suppress traumatic memories. But eventually these hormones decrease, cortisol (the stress hormone) kicks in, and memories come flooding back. Increased cortisol often means a decline in sleep quality.

To return to healthy habits, try this visualization. You may read the instructions all the way through first and then do the exercise; alternatively, you may access a free, guided audio recording at https://www.newharbinger.com/53868.

1. Find a quiet place to sit.

2. Take a few deep breaths.

3. Begin to imagine yourself at the grocery store, walking the aisles in search of whole foods that promote steady blood sugar.

4. Notice the sounds at the store, the smells, and how being there feels in your body.

5. Notice as you pass the coffee, choosing an herbal tea.

6. Next, envision yourself at home, preparing a small healthy meal that supports your body in healing.

7. Then, see yourself getting ready for bed. Do you massage your feet? Listen to quiet music? See yourself climb into bed and easily fall into a restful sleep.

Your Relationship with Exercise

Research shows that exercise is comparable to antidepressants in patients with depression. Physical exercise releases oxytocin, the feel-good hormone, and has been shown to reduce symptoms of anxiety and depression. In addition, exercise can help to strengthen your relationship with your body as you recognize ways it supports your life and health.

Once your doctor has given you the green light for exercise and movement, consider a plan to introduce or reintroduce exercise. What kind of exercise have you enjoyed in the past? Can you make a commitment to reintegrating it into your life, one small step at a time?

Mindful Walking

Mindful walking combines the benefits of mindfulness with the stress-relieving rewards of exercise. This can be a great way to integrate movement if you didn't previously have an exercise practice.

1. Begin by walking slowly.

2. Notice the beginning of your step, the middle, the end, and the pause between steps before your next foot starts moving.

3. Bring your awareness to your feet. Your awareness will drift—to your loss, your mile-long to-do list, the fear that you will never get pregnant again. Notice those thoughts. Then return to your feet.

4. Notice your posture, your swinging arms.

5. Notice the sounds around you, the smells.

6. Notice what you're seeing.

7. Come back to your feet if your mind begins to drift off in thought.

8. Notice the earth beneath you.

9. When you have finished, reflect on your experience in the next prompt.

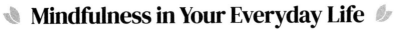 Mindfulness in Your Everyday Life

Share your experience with mindful walking. What other activities can you approach with mindful awareness? They can be as mundane as showering or pushing the grocery cart at the supermarket.

Part V

Stay Open to Support

The despair and heartache that follow a loss may cause you to feel isolated and alone at this vulnerable time. Knowing where and to whom to turn can make all the difference. Expanding your support network can be a helpful step in both mourning and healing from your loss. Reproductive health is a complex issue for many, particularly so in certain locations; finding supports within your family or larger community may be a challenge. You may also determine that social and family support is simply not enough. For many, seeking help from a trained mental health professional can be beneficial. This part of the journal is designed to help you identify supports around you—family, friends, your extended community, trained mental health professionals, among others—to share your hopes and fears in ways that feel safe and authentic.

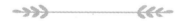

I am learning to ask for help.

⚘ Assessing Your Social Support ⚘

Feeling supported and connected when faced with stressful life challenges improves mental, physical, and emotional health outcomes. Both the quantity and quality of social support may influence well-being when we're grieving. Often, much of the support offered early on by medical providers, friends, and family diminishes quickly, even as the need for support continues.

Share what kinds of support you have received since your loss. Does it feel like enough or not enough? What kind of support would you appreciate more of and from whom?

The Impact of Secrecy in Early Pregnancy

It's common in many societies to wait until the second trimester to announce a pregnancy. This means you may be grieving the loss of your pregnancy and hadn't told anyone you were pregnant. How has your communication about your pregnancy and loss impacted your current emotional state and support from others?

❧ Telling People About Your Loss ❧

It can be challenging to break the news to friends and family members about your loss, but it's incredibly important for your healing that you mobilize a support system. Enlisting a trusted friend, partner, or family member to help disseminate the news can be helpful. How have you communicated with others about your loss so far? Who can help you share the news if you're not up to it now?

Understanding Vulnerability

Vulnerability is "uncertainty, risk, and emotional exposure," according to researcher Brené Brown. It's that shaky feeling you get when you think about doing something out of your comfort zone. Vulnerability is often misunderstood as weakness, when in truth it is the opposite; it takes courage to show up and be seen.

What would it look like for you to be more vulnerable? What brave things might you do and risk being seen?

Practicing Vulnerability

Whether it's sharing your grief with a friend, asking and allowing someone to bring a meal, or reaching out to join a support group, courage is required. And the payoff is worth it—developing deeper connections, feeling less isolated, and being your true authentic self. But how do you get started? The steps below will help you do just that.

Notice the **feeling** of vulnerability in your body. Acknowledge and truly experience any uncomfortable feelings. Don't try to avoid or numb them. Getting used to these sensations will make it easier to sit in vulnerability.

Push yourself outside your comfort zone. What would that be for you? Letting your extended family know you've lost your baby? Telling your friend you can't make their baby shower?

Share your truth. This is the foundational essence of vulnerability. Share your accomplishments, your fears, your love, your feelings of shame and insecurity. Share it all with people you trust.

Practice. Becoming more vulnerable takes practice. Notice your discomfort and then put yourself out there anyway. Eventually, the fear of rejection or judgment will seem insignificant, and following your own heart will become more natural.

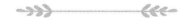

I can accept the emotional support of others.

Identifying the Support You Need

Friends and family may want to help you, but they might not know what to say or do. Brainstorm specific things they can do. For example, ask them to drop off a meal, check in on you by text or phone, watch your other kids, or invite you to get out for a walk. Let them know if you want to talk about your loss or if it's more helpful to have a distraction instead. Write down what kinds of support you'd like. Be as specific as you can, naming who can do which activity.

Sharing with Someone You Trust

Identifying a person who is likely to be supportive and empathic is important. Scan over your world of friends, colleagues, family, and neighbors. Can you identify anyone who has offered you support? Imagine taking a risk and sharing what you're going through. Write about what you hope will happen.

Reaching Out for Support

Now that you've thought about what kind of support you need and who you want to reach out to, it's time to actually do it. Choose one of the people you listed in the Identifying the Support You Need prompt and ask for help. This is an opportunity for you to be brave and practice vulnerability.

Write about what it feels like in your body as you express your needs and speak your truth. What is it like to receive their support? How does it feel to be vulnerable?

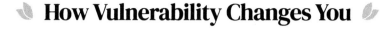 How Vulnerability Changes You

Reflect on what it has been like to practice vulnerability by asking for what you need from others. How does practicing vulnerability impact your relationships? How are things different for you emotionally since you made these efforts?

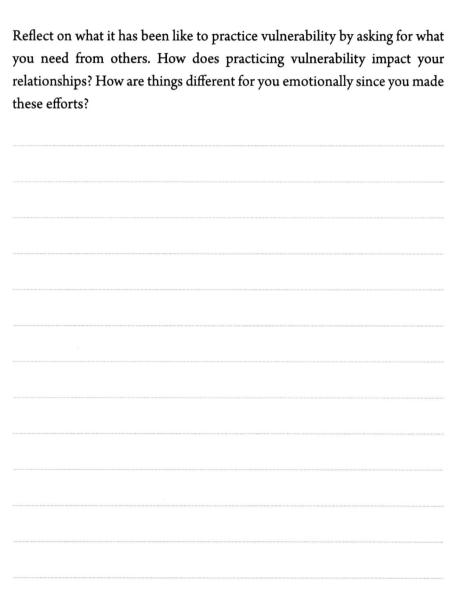

❧ Toxic Positivity Hurts ❧

Toxic positivity is a term for the pressure we might face to have a more "positive" outlook despite the emotional pain we're experiencing. Well-intentioned words of encouragement and positivity from loved ones can sometimes send the message that your sadness and grief are not welcome. Do any of these sound familiar: "At least you know you can get pregnant," "Everything happens for a reason," "You can have more children," "At least it was early"? Instead of soothing your pain, silver lining statements often create greater distance, the opposite of what you may need. Write down any unhelpful words of "support" others have offered since your loss and how they've made you feel.

How to Deal with Toxic Positivity

Despite good intentions, toxic positivity might make you wonder if your grief response is disproportionate to what you've endured or if you're overreacting. This can cause feelings of shame, which often lead to avoidance and isolation from others. It's important to notice this tendency so that you may respond differently.

Brainstorm ways you can respond to someone you care about whose encouragement leaves you feeling disconnected. For example, you might say, "I know you're trying to help, but telling me I can try again makes me feel like you don't understand how much I wanted this baby."

Another approach might be to start the conversation by letting the other person know that you just need an ear and some empathy, and that they don't have to try to fix anything. If it's someone you know casually, like a coworker, you might choose to excuse yourself from the conversation.

Share the unhelpful things people have said to you and how you might respond differently.

Unhelpful encouragement: _____

_____

Your new reply: _____

_____

Unhelpful encouragement: _____

_____

Your new reply: _____

_____

Unhelpful encouragement: _____

_____

Your new reply: _____

_____

🍃 Grieving with Your Partner 🍃

Some couples find that losing a pregnancy or baby brings them closer together. Others may find they drift apart. In heterosexual couples, research shows that most women prefer to talk about their loss, whereas men preferred to deal with it inwardly. How has your loss impacted your connection and relationship with your partner?

Protecting Your Relationship

It's normal for partners to grieve differently from one another. You will each experience a variety of feelings and emotions after a pregnancy or baby loss, and you'll each cope in distinct ways. Assess your relationship in each area. Consider sharing these prompts with your partner and discussing your responses together.

Communication: Are you are able to talk and, perhaps more important, listen to how the other person is feeling? Do you make an effort to understand your partner's perspective?

_____

_____

_____

Intimacy: Do you feel connected to one another? How have you managed to maintain your intimate connection since your loss? Have you discussed how to maintain connection until you're both ready to resume sexual intimacy?

_____

_____

_____

Caretaking: Do you take care of one another? Although you may be grieving differently, there is no one right way. Do you look out for one another and how you're each doing?

Starting a Couple's Journal

It may be difficult to communicate your feelings and needs with your partner. This journal practice allows you to do just that. Start with a commitment of two weeks.

1. Begin with a blank notebook. Lined or unlined is fine.

2. Leave the notebook somewhere easy for both you and your partner to access throughout the day.

3. Write what you feel and what you need each day. It may or may not relate to the loss or to one another.

4. Read what your partner has written and think about how you may or may not be able to support them.

5. If you miss a day, practice self-compassion and begin again tomorrow.

6. After two weeks, check in with your partner about your shared journaling experience. Together, decide if this is something you'd like to continue.

This can be a helpful strategy for opening communication and understanding without having to talk. You might reply offering words of acknowledgment or empathy, letting your partner know you hear what they are going through right now. You may learn what each other is feeling or needing at this moment in time, even if you aren't able to respond right now. Continue journaling together as long as it feels supportive.

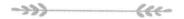

I will get through this; I am not alone.

Finding a Pregnancy or Baby Loss Support Group

Sometimes you just need to talk to someone who's been through what you're going through. A support group can provide a place of community and mutual understanding as you heal from your loss. Use the Resource section at the end of this journal to help you find a virtual or in-person support group. Write down the name, time, and location, and share what it might be like to receive support from others who get what you're going through.

Empowering Yourself to Mute or Unfollow

Social media has a powerful influence on how we feel. Reflect on the impact of your social feeds on your overall well-being. Did you start following pregnancy-related influencers that now make you feel bad? How does it feel when someone you follow announces a pregnancy or birth?

This is a time to offer yourself the care and support you need. Make a list of social media accounts and contacts that leave you feeling down or depressed, or that cause you to compare yourself to others. Which of those can you unfollow or mute?

#ihadamiscarriage, #TFMR, #stillbirth

Social media can also be helpful when used with intention and awareness. Which accounts do you follow that make you laugh, smile, and feel seen?

Check out #ihadamiscarriage, #TFMR, or #stillbirth on Instagram and see what it's like to join a community who shares your struggle. Share three things that you find memorable or inspirational about one of these hashtags.

If social media isn't your thing, you might also read a memoir. Research memoirs and select one that resonates with you. How does reading about others' experiences help decrease the isolation, shame, and stigma of your experience?

❧ Your Network of Support ❧

Reflect on the supports in your life. Support can range from positive emotional energy from a distant relative to a pot of soup from your friend or neighbor. Imagine you are in the middle of this circle of support, surrounded by your family, friends, health care professionals, coworkers, neighbors, and anyone else who has been there for you in the past, whether they are present in your life now or even deceased. Write about the ways you have felt supported by your network.

Part VI

Healing Will Come with Time

As we reach the end of this journal, it is important to remember that neither grief nor healing are linear. The time and energy you have invested in this journal so far—digging deep, reflecting, and practicing new skills—will continue to support you along the road ahead.

This section will help guide you forward. You will begin to explore your goals and dreams for your future as you continue to heal and grow in new directions. Acknowledge yourself for your dedication and effort to your healing and well-being.

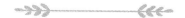

I may never be the same, but what I loved remains part of me.

❧ Disenfranchised Grief ❧

The grief of pregnancy and baby loss is unique in that these losses often aren't recognized by our friends, family, and peers. They are seldom talked about, and with no rituals for these losses they become invisible to others. Without a child, one's identity as a parent is often overlooked, exacerbating feelings of isolation and loneliness. As a result, people may feel less entitled to honor their loss and grieve openly. Dr. Kenneth Doka coined the term *disenfranchised grief,* which encompasses this experience.

How has your community responded to your loss? What feelings come up as you think about disenfranchised grief?

Rituals for Grief

In Western society there are few, if any, rituals specific to pregnancy and baby loss. Some may find comfort in adapting their religious beliefs and holding ceremonies of sorts. Others may find themselves searching, yearning for some way to honor their baby. There is no pressure to do this right away, but many find it helpful to formally acknowledge their loss at some point.

Reflect on the rituals others have embraced. Put a star next to any that resonate with you. Write in other ideas you may be thinking about.

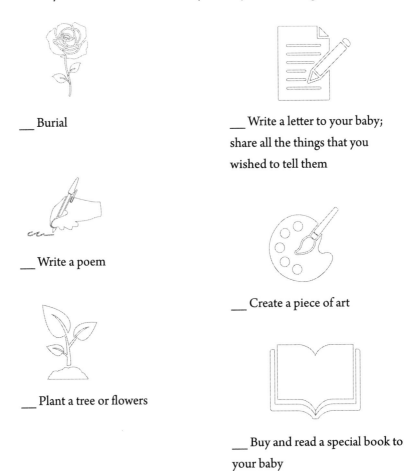

___ Burial

___ Write a letter to your baby; share all the things that you wished to tell them

___ Write a poem

___ Create a piece of art

___ Plant a tree or flowers

___ Buy and read a special book to your baby

___ Adopt rituals from other cultures

___ Create a space in your home that has mementos of your pregnancy and baby

___ Celebrate due dates or birthdates by baking a cake, buying a card, or lighting a candle.

___ Donate to a charity in honor of your baby

___ Get a tattoo

___ Other ....

___ Other ....

___ Other ....

___ Wear a special piece of jewelry

___ Other ....

___ Other ....

Memorializing Your Loss

Making decisions when grieving can be hard. You may yearn for a prescribed ritual that leaves fewer decisions to be made. Rituals are effective in reducing grief because they allow mourners to regain a sense of control at a time when it feels as if they have lost any semblance of control of their lives. Rituals can help to validate your loss, acknowledging that it was real and mattered. Memorializing your loss may provide a way for the memory of your baby to live on with you throughout time. Brainstorm how you'd like to memorialize your pregnancy and loss. Use the list from the previous exercise, research additional ideas, or create your own that resonate.

Important note: If rituals don't feel right to you, please don't do them to appease others. Memorializing is a personal expression meant to help you in finding peace within.

Processing Grief in Small Bites

Identifying your feelings and sharing your story in small pieces over time are ways to process your grief. Retelling helps to move the trauma from an experience that's relived over and over again in the present to being a memory from the past. With this in mind, browse this journal and complete any unanswered prompts that could benefit your healing, or revisit ones that you found cathartic. Try a practice or exercise that you had skipped. If you're not ready, note the page numbers below so you can go back when you are ready.

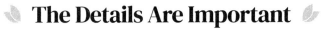 The Details Are Important

Telling the details of your story to someone you trust can facilitate healing. Even the graphic details of blood and physical pain. If you experienced a medical emergency, saw the fetus or baby, experienced feelings of powerlessness—these details are part of your story and deserve to be told and heard by others when you're ready. Reflect on what it was like to share these details. If you haven't yet shared these parts, explore what has stopped you.

Going at Your Own Pace

There is no timeline for healing. This includes your readiness to try again for another baby. You may not know when or if you will try again. You may already be trying. Others may ask when you'll be ready. They may suggest you try again to help you move forward.

Wherever you are in the process, allow yourself to take your time. Write about where you are right now.

....

....

....

....

....

....

....

....

....

--->>>———————<<<---

I accept the natural ups and downs of life.

Affirmations for Healing

Affirmations are positive statements used to challenge negative, depressing, or anxiety-producing thoughts and beliefs. Affirmations can be a powerful way to influence your thinking patterns, behavioral habits, health, and moods. Throughout this journal I've included a few affirmations. Hopefully you have found these supportive.

Now it's your turn to create personalized affirmations. Write down at least ten positive affirmations that resonate with you.

A few tips on creating affirmations:

- Write them in the present or future tense.

- Start with "I" or "My."

- Keep them short and positive.

- Include an emotion, for example, "I feel [emotion]" or "I am [emotion] about…"

- Reframe a negative thought you have about yourself to its positive, counteracting opposite, for instance, "I am brave" instead of "I am scared."

- Make sure it is believable. If you come up with an affirmation that's difficult for you to believe, reframe it as "I am open to…" or "I am willing to believe I could…"

1. _____

_____

2.

3.

4.

5.

6.

7.

8.

9.

10.

Affirming Your Courage to Heal

Practicing affirmations fires up your neural pathways and makes changes to those areas of the brain that reinforce happiness. They can train your mind to think positive thoughts about yourself. They have even been shown to lower stress and rumination, which contribute to depression and anxiety.

Refer to the list of affirmations you created in the previous exercise, then follow the steps to allow your affirmations a bolder presence in your life.

1. Write your favorite affirmations on sticky notes to place around your home.

2. As you place the notes, take three slow breaths as you repeat the affirmation to yourself.

3. Whenever you see the sticky notes, pause, and take a breath as you affirm yourself.

🍃 Fear of Moving On 🍃

You may fear a future pregnancy and the risk of another loss. Or perhaps you're afraid that trying to conceive again means you will forget your pregnancy and baby. Wanting to grow your family yet struggling with fear are common yet complicated feelings people grapple with after a pregnancy loss.

Practicing self-compassion, share three things you can say to yourself in response to your fear. Be kind and gentle with yourself. Talk to yourself as you would a friend.

1. _____

   _____

2. _____

   _____

3. _____

   _____

A New Baby Is Not Always a Solution

For some, having a healthy baby after a loss brings relief and feelings of joy. For others, a new baby can trigger the pain of loss. Reaching out for additional help now, or knowing what resources are available for future support, can make a difference on your journey of deciding when or if you want to try again.

For starters, find Postpartum Support International online. Write down three names from its provider directory who are in your area. Next, jot down some ideas of what you might like to discuss with them. Most therapists included have expertise supporting people prenatally and after loss, however, feel free to ask about their experience directly. The credential "PMH-C" after a name stands for Perinatal Mental Health Certified; it indicates that the therapist or psychiatrist has obtained the highest level of training available in perinatal mental health.

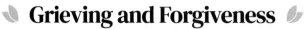 Grieving and Forgiveness

Sometimes the most compassionate thing we can do is forgive. Forgiveness involves grieving before letting go of feelings like anger, fear, or guilt. It requires that you are open to whatever emotions you feel. Perhaps your friends, family, or partner have let you down. Maybe it was a doctor. Maybe you don't feel good about the way you responded to something. This isn't about judgment but rather about recognizing the sadness and pain you carry, and the grudges you may be holding on to that do not serve you.

What do you need to grieve in order to let go and forgive? Consider writing a letter to process your feelings and experience; you can choose later whether to send it.

Forgiveness Practice

Forgiveness is making the conscious choice to release yourself from the burden, pain, and stress of holding on to resentment. It's important to give yourself permission to acknowledge and honor the pain that's very real for you. Only then can you let it go. Let's try this now.

1. Think about what or who has caused the pain that you've been unwilling to forgive. Feel the pain you still carry as you hold tightly to your unwillingness to forgive.

2. Now, observe what emotion is present. Is it anger, guilt, resentment, sadness?

3. Notice physically what you feel. Is it tension, heaviness? Note where you feel it in your body.

4. Bring awareness to your thoughts. Are they hateful, spiteful, or something else?

5. As you focus on the pain you have endured and the hurt that lives inside you, ask yourself, "Who is suffering? Have I carried this burden long enough? Am I willing to forgive?"

6. If the answer is no, that's okay. Some wounds need more time than others to heal.

7. If you are ready to let it go now, as you breathe in, silently repeat: "I acknowledge the pain."

8. As you breathe out, repeat: "I am forgiving and releasing this burden from my heart and mind."

9. Continue this process for as long as it feels supportive to you.

Your Reproductive Story Continues

You may notice your feelings vacillate—you may have one foot in the past and one leaning into the future. You have been forever changed by your loss, yet your reproductive story is incomplete and will continue to unfold as time marches on. There's no preset timeline and no shoulds. Honor the ebb and flow of your feelings.

How has your story changed since you started this journal? What have you learned about yourself? Pay attention to your body as well as your heart. Offer yourself words of compassion as you reflect on your story.

I am hopeful; I am capable; I am strong.

Even Just One Therapy Session Can Help

Research shows that just one counseling session following a pregnancy or baby loss can impact one's psychological well-being. Discussing traumatic events like pregnancy loss with someone objective or who isn't part of your daily life can be helpful. Consider the various options for support: one-on-one therapy, group therapy, text or virtual therapy, free social media groups. Imagine what it would be like to seek additional support for your grief. What would it be like to talk with someone you don't know about your loss?

Reconnecting with Your Strengths

You may feel disconnected from the person you were before your loss. Reconnecting with parts of yourself that previously existed and made you strong and unique can support your healing. Are there things you once loved about yourself that seem lost? What made you feel most empowered? Make a list of your innate strengths and passions, whether that's home design, cooking, nature, or planning an incredible trip. Are you detail oriented, patient, loving, social justice minded? Describe your positive traits and pastimes.

The Emotional Calendar

It's common to anticipate your due date or the anniversary of your loss with some trepidation. Other events are likely to trigger feelings of grief and loss as well, the first year in particular. What dates or holidays do you anticipate may be difficult for you? Who can you count on to support you during these times?

Your Journaling Reflections

Using a guided journal, such as this one, can bring new thoughts and feelings to the surface. You may discover you're worried about something you didn't know was disturbing you until you wrote it down. You may notice new patterns. You may find that writing helps you feel more in charge of your life, and you may discover new strengths you didn't realize you had. What have you learned through writing and rereading your journal?

Moving Forward

Grieving your loss and coming to terms with the unexpected requires courage to continuously show up to what is present. In order to adapt and move forward, it's important to bring self-compassion to the forefront of your mind. You may need to remind yourself that you didn't do anything to cause this and that you will feel better if you can accept your loss. Acknowledging your feelings and determining what you can control will help. Creating and sticking to an action plan to eat nourishing food, get adequate sleep and fresh air, find ways to move your body that feel good, and socialize in person or virtually are key.

Write down specific ways you can ensure self-care remains part of your routine.

What are three things you'd like to continue or start doing each day?

1. _____

2. _____

3. _____

Each week?

1. _____

2. _____

3. _____

Which friends or family members can you enlist to help you make time and stick to your plan?

1. _____

2. _____

3. _____

Small Steps Forward

You've put in a great deal of effort toward healing after your loss. My hope is that you've started to feel better physically, emotionally, and mentally. Maintaining this toolbox of strategies and your support system is crucial to navigating this unexpected and traumatic loss.

Grief and loss change us in countless ways. We are challenged to oscillate between intense sorrow and unanticipated growth, as you've explored throughout this journal. Going forward, know it's normal to experience sadness and grief. They are an inevitable part of the journey, not an indicator that anything is wrong.

It's also expected that one moment you are steeped in grief, missing your baby, and the next moment navigating your return to work. This ebb and flow between loss and assimilation of this new part of your identity is normal. You will be confronted with new opportunities to adapt and accept your evolving reproductive story as your future unfolds and you figure out how to live with your loss. Leaning on others and using the new strategies you have practiced can help you manage challenging moments as they arise.

Note which journal exercises have been particularly useful for you and return to them when needed. Acknowledge your vulnerability, strength, and courage, which have been called on to address this challenging, unanticipated, and unwelcome loss. Recognize your resilience. Consult the Resources section of this journal for books, websites, and more that can offer you additional support today and in the future.

Finally, acknowledge yourself for your hard work. I wish you the very best as you continue your journey.

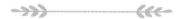

I am strong, confident, and resilient,
and I am more than my grief.

Acknowledgments

It takes a tremendous amount of courage to reach out for help in healing from a pregnancy or baby loss. I'm grateful to my clients and others who have trusted me with their stories and allowed me to support them through the pain and despair of their traumatic grief.

I am grateful to my husband and children for their unwavering patience and encouragement. I must also acknowledge the losses we endured and the passion and compassion that grew from that grief into my most enriching work—and now this journal.

And to my own former therapist, Dr. J. J., who supported me through some of the darkest moments and helped me find my way here to this moment.

Resources

Information, Education, and Support

EMDRIA is a professional association for practitioners trained in eye movement desensitization and reprocessing (EMDR), an evidence-based trauma therapy. EMDRIA hosts a provider directory.

https://www.emdria.org

Ending a Wanted Pregnancy offers access to a private Facebook support group and an online space for sharing and reading others' stories.

https://www.endingawantedpregnancy.com

Miscarriage Association supports those affected by miscarriage, molar pregnancy, or ectopic pregnancy.

https://www.miscarriageassociation.org.uk

Postpartum Support International (PSI) offers free peer support groups for parents who have experienced miscarriage, stillbirth, TFMR, and infant death, as well as various groups for pregnancy and parenting after loss. PSI hosts a provider directory.

https://www.postpartum.net

Return to Zero: HOPE provides support, resources, and community for all people who have experienced loss during the journey to parenthood. It hosts a provider directory.

https://www.rtzhope.org

Share Pregnancy and Infant Loss Support offers information, education, and resources in support of bereaved families.

https://nationalshare.org

What's Your Grief? provides community, support, resources, and education for those grieving and those looking to support someone who's grieving.

https://www.whatsyourgrief.com

Mindfulness

Dr. Arielle Schwartz
Free trauma-informed guided yoga
https://drarielleschwartz.com

UCSD Center for Mindfulness
Free guided meditations
https://cih.ucsd.edu/mindfulness

UCLA Mindful Awareness Research Center
Free guided meditations
https://www.uclahealth.org/marc

Kristin Neff
Free guided self-compassion practices
https://www.self-compassion.org

Mindfulness Apps

Calm

Expectful

Headspace

Insight Timer

Books

Empty Cradle, Broken Heart: Surviving the Death of Your Baby
by Deborah L. Davis

Emotional Agility: Get Unstuck, Embrace Change and Thrive in Work and Life by Susan David

Healing from Reproductive Trauma: A Workbook for Survivors of Traumatic Infertility Journeys, Pregnancies and Births by Bethany Warren

I Had a Miscarriage: A Memoir, a Movement by Jessica Zucker

I Love You Still: A Memorial Baby Book by Margaret Scofield

It's OK That You're Not OK: Meeting Grief and Loss in a Culture That Doesn't Understand by Megan Devine

Not Broken: An Approachable Guide to Miscarriage and Recurrent Pregnancy Loss by Lora Shahine, MD

The Baby Loss Guide: Practical and Compassionate Support with a Day-by-Day Resource to Navigate the Path of Grief by Zoe Clark-Coates

The Burden of Choice: Collected Stories from Parents Facing a Diagnosis of Abnormalities During Pregnancy by Georgina Pearson

The Miscarriage Map: What to Expect When You Are No Longer Expecting by Sunita Osborn

What God Is Honored Here?: Writings on Miscarriage and Infant Loss by and for Native Women and Women of Color by Shannon Gibney

When Hello Means Goodbye by Paul Kirk and Pat Schwiebert

Books for Children

We Were Gonna Have a Baby, But We Had an Angel Instead by Pat Schwiebert, illustrated by Taylor Bills

Something Happened by Cathy Blanford

My Sibling Still: For Those Who've Lost a Sibling to Miscarriage, Stillbirth, and Infant Death by Megan Lacourrege, illustrated by Joshua Wichterich

Instagram

@ihadamiscarriage

@mainstreammiscarriage

@miscarriagemomma

@stilllovedbabies

@tfmrmamas

@sistersinloss

@stilllovedbabies

@theworstgirlgangever

@tfmrpsychologist

References

American College of Obstetricians and Gynecologists. "Early Pregnancy Loss: FAQs." Accessed October 27, 2023. https://www.acog.org/womens-health/faqs/early-pregnancy-loss.

Bardos, J., D. Hercz, J. Friedenthal, S. A. Missmer, and Z. Williams. 2015. "A National Survey on Public Perceptions of Miscarriage." *Obstetrics & Gynecology* 125(6): 1313–1320. https://doi.org/10.1097/aog.0000000000000859.

Brach, T. 2011. "Working with Difficulties: The Blessings of RAIN." Tara Brach (blog), July 1. https://www.tarabrach.com/rain-workingwithdifficulties.

Brown, B. 2022. *Atlas of the Heart: Mapping Meaningful Connection and the Language of Human Experience.* New York: Random House.

Cacciatore, J., K. Thieleman, R. Fretts, and L. Barnes Jackson. 2021. "What Is Good Grief Support? Exploring the Actors and Actions in Social Support after Traumatic Grief." *PLOS ONE* 16(5): e0252324. https://doi.org/10.1371/journal.pone.0252324.

David, S. A. 2017. *Emotional Agility: Get Unstuck, Embrace Change, and Thrive in Work and Life.* New York: Avery.

Devine, M. 2021. *How to Carry What Can't Be Fixed: A Journal for Grief.* Boulder, CO: Sounds True.

Doka, K. J. 2002. *Disenfranchised Grief: New Directions, Challenges, and Strategies for Practice.* Champaign, IL: Research Press.

Emery, R., and J. Coan. 2010. "Why Is Talking with Gestures Easier Than Talking Without Them?" *Scientific American Mind*, March 1. https://doi.org/10.1038/scientificamericanmind0310-72.

Ezrin, S. 2021. "5 Poses to Inspire More Self-Love, Less Self Smack-Talk." *Yoga Journal*, September 2. https://www.yogajournal.com/practice/yoga-sequences/yoga-for-self-love-a-5-pose-home-practice.

Gordon, J. S. 2021. *Transforming Trauma: The Path to Hope and Healing*. San Francisco: HarperOne.

Harris, R. 2019. *ACT Made Simple: An Easy-To-Read Primer on Acceptance and Commitment Therapy*, 2nd ed. Oakland, CA: New Harbinger Publications.

Hasson, G. 2017. *Confidence Pocketbook: Little Exercises for a Self-Assured Life*. Chichester, UK: Capstone.

Heissel, A., D. Heinen, L. L. Brokmeier, N. Skarabis, M. Kangas, D. Vancampfort, B. Stubbs, et al. 2023. "Exercise as Medicine for Depressive Symptoms? A Systematic Review and Meta-Analysis with Meta-Regression." *British Journal of Sports Medicine* 57(16): 1049–1057. https://doi.org/10.1136/bjsports-2022-106282.

Jaffe, J. 2017. "Reproductive Trauma: Psychotherapy for Pregnancy Loss and Infertility Clients from a Reproductive Story Perspective." *Psychotherapy* 54(4): 380–385. https://doi.org/10.1037/pst0000125.

Jarero, I., and L. Artigas. 2023. "The EMDR Therapy Butterfly Hug Method for Self-Administered Bilateral Stimulation." *Research Gate*. https://www.researchgate.net/publication/340280320.

Kersting, A., and B. Wagner. 2012. "Complicated Grief After Perinatal Loss." *Dialogues in Clinical Neuroscience* 14(2): 187–194. https://doi.org/10.31887/dcns.2012.14.2/akersting.

Kircanski, K., M. D. Lieberman, and M. G. Craske. 2012. "Feelings into Words." *Psychological Science* 23(10): 1086–1091. https://doi.org/10.1177/0956797612443830.

Koch, L. 2018. "The One Muscle That Does Not Need Strengthening." *Core Awareness*, April 3. https://coreawareness.com/the-one-muscle-that-does-not-need-strengthening.

Logan, M. 2020. *Self-Love Workbook for Women: Release Self-Doubt, Build Self-Compassion, and Embrace Who You Are*. Emeryville, CA: Rockridge Press.

Maagh, L. C., E. Quinlan, S. Vicary, S. Schilder, and C. Carey. 2023. "Self-Compassion and Mental Health in Australian Women Who Have Experienced Pregnancy Loss." *Illness, Crisis & Loss* 0(0). https://doi.org/10.1177/10541373221150326.

Neff, K., and C. K. Germer. 2018. *The Mindful Self-Compassion Workbook: A Proven Way to Accept Yourself, Build Inner Strength, and Thrive.* New York: Guilford Press.

Neimeyer, R. A., D. Klass, and M. R. Dennis. 2014. "A Social Constructionist Account of Grief: Loss and the Narration of Meaning." *Death Studies* 38: 485–498. http://doi.org/10.1080/07481187.2014.913454.

Neugebauer, R. 1997. "Major Depressive Disorder in the 6 Months after Miscarriage." *JAMA* 277(5): 383–388. https://doi.org/10.1001/jama.1997.03540290035029.asaaaasssssssssssss2s.

Pennebaker, J. W., and J. M. Smyth. 2016. *Opening Up by Writing It Down: How Expressive Writing Improves Health and Eases Emotional Pain.* New York: Guilford Press.

Raes, F., E. Pommier, K. D. Neff, and D. Van Gucht. 2011. "Construction and Factorial Validation of a Short Form of the Self-Compassion Scale." *Clinical Psychology & Psychotherapy* 18: 250–255. https://doi.org/10.1002/cpp.702.

Swanson, K. M., Z. A. Karmali, S. H. Powell, and F. Pulvermakher. 2003. "Miscarriage Effects on Couples' Interpersonal and Sexual Relationships During the First Year after Loss: Women's Perceptions." *Psychosomatic Medicine* 65(5): 902–910. https://doi.org/10.1097/01.psy.0000079381.58810.84.

Wenzel, A. 2015. *Coping with Infertility, Miscarriage, and Neonatal Loss: Finding Perspective and Creating Meaning.* Washington, DC: American Psychological Association.

Rachel Rabinor, LCSW, is a licensed clinical social worker providing individual and group therapy in San Diego, CA, and virtually throughout the state. Rabinor specializes in reproductive mental health, trauma-based therapy, and perinatal mental health. She is a member of the Mental Health Professional Group (MHPG) of the American Society for Reproductive Medicine (ASRM), the Pregnancy Loss and Infant Death Association (PLIDA), RESOLVE, EMDRIA, and the Postpartum Health Alliance. Rabinor is author of *The Postpartum Depression Journal*, and has coauthored two chapters on "Fertility Counseling with Groups" in the second edition of *Fertility Counseling*.

Foreword writer **Janet Jaffe, PhD**, is cofounder and director of the Center for Reproductive Psychology in San Diego, CA, and is coauthor of *Unsung Lullabies: Understanding and Coping with Infertility*.

MORE BOOKS from
NEW HARBINGER PUBLICATIONS

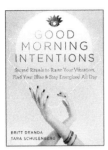
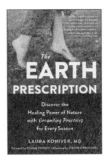
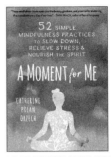
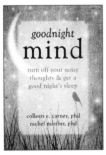
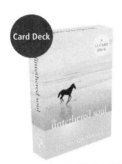
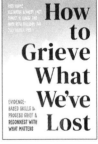